As We Think...
So We Age

Other Books by Geri Marr Burdman

Health Aspects of Aging (with Ruth Brewer, Eds.)

Healthful Aging

Joyful Aging

Search for Significance: Finding Meaning in Times of Change, Challenge, and Chaos

The Boy Who Ate Poi (with Chaison Kalili-Burdman)

As We Think...
So We Age—
Exploring Pathways to
Meaningful Aging

Geri Marr Burdman, Ph.D.

GeroWise® Books
A Division of GeroWise® International

Interior design & layout: PurposeResearch.com

Cover design: Roberto Burdman

Editors: Charles McLafferty, Jr. & Kate Robinson

Cover photo: "Path through a colorful garden"
National Arboretum, Washington, DC
Image used under license from Shutterstock.com

ISBN: 978-0-692-44021-6

To My Sons
Robert Peter
and
Ethan David
and
To My Global Family

Contents

Introduction

"Let me stand in my age
with all its waters flowing round me."

—MARGARET FULLER

Sipping an espresso at a used bookstore one drizzly Seattle afternoon, I browsed shelves teeming with books of all genres. Suddenly, I stumbled upon *Healthful Aging*, a college textbook I authored over two decades ago. I recognized its deep green cover with that luminous sunlit background, and smiled inwardly, thinking, "who turned my book in for cash?"

I stopped browsing and began reminiscing, remembering the invitations that book brought me to present seminars and workshops on health promotion and aging. I mused about its readers; it was obviously well read by more than one gerontology student. There were notations throughout, alongside those ubiquitous neon yellow highlights that students seem to love. As I perused the notes, a large

calligraphic-like script leapt off the very last page:
"As we think… so we age."

I have no idea who the reader was, but those six words capture the essence of a keynote that I deeply embrace and try to communicate through my work and in my life. Thank you, whoever you are! I would only add that our *attitudes* also determine our experience of aging.

So, you may wonder, why would anyone view aging as a product of thoughts or even of attitudes?

Growing up in rural Minnesota, my grandfather was my hero. I did not really think of him as old or even aging; he was just "Gramps," a steady presence whose unconditional love provided bedrock throughout my childhood. In retrospect, I am aware that my grandfather was really my first teacher of *gerontology*: the study of aging. Grandpa Marr had seen his share of sorrow during the Great Depression of the 1930s; he lost his farm in southwestern Minnesota followed by the sudden death of his beloved wife, Emily, my grandmother.

Yet, growing up, I knew nothing of the hardships he'd endured. As a child, I cherished summertime with Gramps. His old rust-colored Nash was always at the ready to drive me to fill jugs of springwater from a bubbling brook on the outskirts of town or to view the setting sun from a grassy knoll near my grandmother's gravesite.

I remember Gramps as a gentle soul. I never heard him utter an unkind word. Over the years, I've learned that many who have been drawn to the field of gerontology can vividly recall extraordinary relationships with elders, often a grandparent. I had no idea of the tumult my grandfather's family experienced until I recently came upon a faded journal with a few tattered pages of sketchily penned family history. My grandfather was born a twin. He and his brother, Nate, were the last of 15 children his mother birthed in rural Wisconsin. Three of those 15 succumbed to "fevers" one harsh winter before the twins—Ethan and Nathan—arrived. Gramps was quiet and contemplative, a man of few words rarely prone to display emotion. I often saw him deep in reflection; he appeared to be reminiscing, engaged in what we now call "life review." No doubt he was recalling past events and trying to make sense of it all. Had I known then what I know now about the critical importance of life review in later years, I would have asked more questions. And I would certainly have listened more carefully!

Gramps always encouraged me to follow my dreams. From an early age, I regaled him with my plans to study nursing and to see the world, in that order. He listened patiently and usually quietly responded: "Snookie, you can do whatever you set your mind to."

I did study nursing and the same year that I passed my Minnesota state board exams to become a registered nurse, the Peace Corps was born. What a sublime coincidence! Accepted into Peace Corps training in early 1962, a mere three months later I found myself in the heart of South America: Sucre, Bolivia. Serving as a Peace Corps Volunteer in Bolivia opened doors I'd never dreamed possible. The experience ignited my passion for global health work and helped shape my worldview in ways that I will explore with you in this book.

It was in Bolivia, and several years later in Puerto Rico, that I began to seriously ponder questions about the relationship between one's attitude and the process of aging. I lived with a four-generation family in Bolivia; in Puerto Rico, I lived right next door to a four-generation household. Yes, four generations under the same roof! Up close and personal glimpses of intergenerational dynamics pointed me in the direction of my life's work. During the two years in Bolivia followed by nearly seven years in Puerto Rico, innumerable cross-generational and cross-cultural interactions fueled my curiosity about meaningful aging.

When I began studying for a master's degree at the University of Puerto Rico in 1968, I had no idea that gerontology was even a field of study. But I jumped at a life-changing opportunity when I learned that Dr. Viktor Frankl was traveling to the Island of Puerto Rico from his home in Vienna, Austria to present a series of seminars. Yes, Viktor Frankl, the world-renowned author of the book listed by the United States Library of Congress as one of the 10 most influential books ever written: *Man's Search for Meaning*. It was directly from Professor Frankl that I learned vital lessons about unconditional meaningfulness across the lifespan—lessons that opened portals to understanding and that continue to inform my attitude about aging and about life itself. Profoundly impacted by his work, I vowed to pursue further education that would allow me to immerse myself in the interdisciplinary study of gerontology.

A few years later, when I landed in verdant Eugene, Oregon to study for a Ph.D., I was welcomed by two exemplary University of Oregon professors who not only understood but also enthusiastically supported and nurtured my penchant for gerontological and cross-cultural studies. Drs. Warren Smith and Frances Scott guided me onto a pathway that I have pursued for over four decades. The

University's health education and gerontology programs offered unique opportunities to combine my passions: community health and the study of aging. With the support of Fran Scott, a pioneer in the field who directed one of the first interdisciplinary academic centers on gerontology in the United States, I was awarded an Administration on Aging scholarship to complete my doctoral work. Simultaneously, I received a graduate teaching fellowship as I was mentored by Warren Smith, whose extensive knowledge of global health motivated me to explore international work opportunities. Both of my mentors became dear friends, and I corresponded with each of them well into their retirement years as they continued to express keen interest in my work. Shortly before passing from this earth plane at age 90, Dr. Smith sent me a personally inscribed book he had just completed: *World Health: Historical and Current Perspectives.* I treasure his gift; he was an extraordinary mentor whose unfailing kindness has served as a role model for me and countless others.

The lives and deeds of these and scores of other "way-showers" who have influenced the direction of my life and my personal journey toward meaningful aging are featured in each chapter of this book.

Look to this Day

Look to this day,
For it is life,
The very life of life.
In its brief course lie all
The realities and truths of existence,
The joy of growth,
The splendor of action,
The glory of power—
For yesterday is but a dream
And tomorrow is only a vision.
But today, well lived,
Makes every yesterday a memory of happiness
And every tomorrow a vision of hope.
Look well, therefore, to this day.

—SANSKRIT PROVERB

Reflections:

One
Find Meaning in Each New Day

"When we are no longer able to change a situation,
we are challenged to change ourselves."

—VIKTOR FRANKL

In Pursuit of Meaning

Dashing between classes on the hibiscus-laden campus
of the University of Puerto Rico in the late 1960s,
I paused to scan some ads on a cluttered bulletin board.
Among "rooms for rent," "rides to Ponce," and a swarm of
other announcements, a handwritten note caught my eye:

> Dr. Viktor E. Frankl
> Holocaust Survivor, Founder of Logotherapy
> The Third Viennese School of Psychotherapy
> Presenting a Seminar for Faculty and
> Graduate Students Today at 4 P. M.

I seized the opportunity to attend that seminar, but little did I know I would walk into a life-changing event. As I paused at the entryway, I sensed a stillness—an almost sacrosanct atmosphere—in the classroom. I'd arrived just in time to catch a glimpse of the bespectacled, sprightly Viktor Frankl striding confidently toward the mahogany podium as a palpable hush came over the room. Without hesitation, Dr. Frankl began speaking in a serene, resolute voice about his life's work and the unspeakable suffering he and his loved ones had endured at the hands of the Nazis. His wife, mother, father, brother, sister-in-law, and mother-in-law—along with six million Jews and fifteen million others—perished in the concentration camps.

I became transfixed as Viktor Frankl explained that he was already writing and lecturing on what he termed "logotherapy" years before World War II. He had studied extensively with Drs. Sigmund Freud and Alfred Adler, founders of two Viennese schools of psychotherapy of his era. However, Dr. Frankl went on to say that while he respected these great teachers, he differentiated his philosophy and psychology from theirs.

What riveted my attention that day was his calm demeanor and unwavering conviction that humans are not merely destined to "pursue pleasure," as Freud taught, or to "seek power," as Adler proposed. "There is a greater motivating force behind all human behavior and that is the search for meaning," Frankl maintained. Furthermore, he insisted that the motivating element in life cannot be the mere pursuit of success or happiness: "these must come as by-products!"

Now, you may be asking: What, then, does this have to do with aging? Or, for that matter, "as we think... so we age?"

Discovering purpose and meaning at each stage of life is essential to aging healthfully. Yet that very word *aging* is fraught with misconceptions, fear, and dread. News media feed us daily doses of the daunting challenges facing older adults as well as their families and communities. Repeatedly, we are reminded that the population of older people is growing at the fastest rate in recorded history. Aging affects every nation; global demographic changes are altering the social and economic nature of our entire planet. Indeed, a person plucked from a mere century ago and set down in today's world would be struck, not only by the sheer number of older adults, but by their visibility and imprint on society.

Searching for a meaningful anchor can seem an onerous task in today's world of uncertainty. Yet a path toward a wholesome image—and a positive experience—of aging is accessible regardless of what is happening in our lives. That path calls us to be vigilant; it is a bold invitation to embrace an attitudinal shift, to step into a new paradigm.

When I met Viktor Frankl in Puerto Rico over four decades ago, I was a curious and eager graduate student pursuing a master's degree in counseling, but I had no idea that his message would affect me so profoundly. I was immediately struck by the absolute absence of rancor in his voice.

When Frankl quoted the words of Frederick Nietzsche—"He who has a why to live for can endure almost any how"—I felt compelled to scribble a few key words on my notepad. I attempted to comprehend how this man could possibly maintain a positive attitude given the magnitude of his personal losses.

Frankl simply described the core of logotherapy as "meaning-based psychotherapy." Reflecting on his own heart-rending experiences, he unequivocally stated that humans have the capacity to suffer courageously, even to bring good out of unavoidable adversity. Viktor Frankl insisted that the ability to choose one's attitude toward any situation is irrevocable.

Our Search for Significance Across the Lifespan

Viktor Frankl, whose life work focused on helping people find meaning regardless of age or social condition, insisted: "We must never forget that we may find meaning in life even when confronted with a seemingly hopeless situation, when facing a fate that cannot be changed. When we are no longer able to change a situation, we are challenged to change ourselves."

Frankl also addressed a common human malady: alienation, a sense of estrangement or abandonment, of not belonging, of not fitting in. In today's world, this feeling of inner emptiness takes a huge toll on health and quality of life; often it manifests as depression or despair. He called it an *existential vacuum*.

A search for meaning is a universal longing among humans; we yearn for a purpose worthy of our efforts. When we are engaged in whatever gives us a sense of significance, a reason to get out of bed and organize the day, the quality of our days is bound to improve.

Frankl taught that portals to meaning may be found:
- by doing a deed,
- through loving, and
- by choosing the attitude we take toward adversity.

Reaching out and helping another is "doing a deed." There are thousands of ways to touch another through simple acts of kindness. We need only look around. Opportunities abound!

Gaining a keen appreciation of nature, a work of art, or the essence of another human is integral to developing a meaningful attitude toward life itself. "Loving" refers to that dimension which allows us to see one another with a heart of compassion.

When faced with a situation that cannot be changed, such as the death of a family member, disruptions in work or home, financial instability, divorce, illness, or other major upheavals, we are given an ultimate opportunity to actualize the highest value, to fulfill the deepest meaning—the "meaning of suffering." What matters above all is the attitude we take: how we face events and circumstances that may be completely beyond our control. Our quality of life depends upon our ability to shift gears, to accept—and even to transform—life's challenges and vicissitudes, no matter how arduous the process.

Viktor Frankl's message left an imprint on my heart that remains to this day. Profoundly moved by the gentleness of his presence and his compassion, I vividly recall his closing remarks from that seminar in Puerto Rico: the moment he exhorted us to "Listen to the person in the street. He or she may be your teacher!"

I felt a distinct resonance with Frankl's powerful words, unlike anything I had ever experienced. A shift in my conscious awareness was occurring and I intuitively knew I should pay attention! Needing to be alone for a while, I made a beeline across campus to a tiny alcove encased by multicolored bougainvillea adjacent to the library. As I sat in stunned silence, I jotted another note to myself: *Take time, listen: Who are your real teachers?*

My work from that day forward has been to listen, to learn, and to share the wisdom of teachers I encounter along the way. Over the years, global health work assignments have taken me to many parts of the world.

I find great teachers in the most unlikely situations and locales. Listening to the person in the street does yield amazing lessons!

From Quechua women of Bolivia to Maori elders in New Zealand to health workers of Kenya to university students in Grenada to spiritual healers of Bali to indigenous midwives in Guatemala to grandmothers raising children in Hawaii, all—and many more—have been my teachers.

I have noted repeatedly that the people who are most solidly grounded, regardless of age or circumstances, are focused on others. Connected with others through mutual need, these individuals tend to share some common characteristics: an acceptance of responsibility for themselves and their own actions and deeds, flexibility and resilience in the face of change and adversity, a capacity to accept sorrow as well as joy, and a sense of community and responsibility toward neighbors and family alike.

"Between stimulus and response
there is a space.
In that space is our power
to choose our response.
In our response
lies our growth and our freedom."

—VIKTOR E. FRANKL

"You cannot control what happens to you,
but you can control your attitude toward
what happens to you,
and in that,
you will be mastering change
rather than allowing it to master you."

—VIKTOR E. FRANKL

"The journey
of a thousand miles
begins
with a single step."

—LAO TZU

Reflections:

Two
Recognize Your Unique Place in the Web of the World

"In the midst of winter,
I discovered that there was, within me,
an Invincible Summer."

—ALBERT CAMUS

After accepting an invitation to speak at a conference near Sydney, Australia, years ago, I pondered with considerable trepidation the topic I was asked to address: *Dealing with Despair: Our Search for Significance.* I clearly remember Faye Cameron, the conference coordinator, introducing me to an audience comprised largely of health and social service providers. After graciously reciting my degrees, affiliations, and sundry other qualifications, she posed three stark questions seeking answers to vexing global dilemmas:

- Why are depression and despair so prevalent in our world today?
- Is there some gnawing inner emptiness?
- Are there antidotes for despair?

Now I knew why I felt such hesitation about tackling this vast and daunting topic! But I agreed to share some lessons I've learned from sojourners on my path. I chose to emphasize that the search for purpose and meaning—significance—is a universal longing. It is our deep desire to make sense of our lives in the midst of change... and, yes, even in despair.

Depression and despair are not new on the horizon. For the past couple of centuries, depression, or melancholy as it was once called, has figured prominently in the lives of such noteworthy individuals as the Russian novelist Leo Tolstoy, German social scientist Max Weber, American psychologist William James, and English playwright and essayist Samuel Johnson, among scores of others. Indeed, the condition called depression grew in prevalence over the course of the 20th century and has increased to pandemic (worldwide) proportions. And this malady strikes all levels of society; it affects women and men of all ages.

In recent years, numerous media outlets have focused on the toll of depression in the workplace and in society at large. The roles of gender and genetic factors, as well as pharmacological and counseling interventions, are subjects of continuous study. And the use of medication in the treatment and management of depression is increasingly prevalent. Yet there is a whole lot more to the picture!

As I often do, I invited audience participation as I reframed the first question raised by the conference coordinator: "Why are symptoms of despair and depression seen so often in our communities today?"

Immediately that query brought forth a familiar audience response: "Because people don't have good support networks, they are disconnected from family and friends, distant from that which gives them grounding."

Suddenly, as if a spigot had burst, participants poured forth stories of neighbors isolated at home, distant from relatives and no longer able to drive… tales of loneliness, depression, family conflicts, caregiver burnout, and so much more. We could have been anywhere in the world; I've heard these challenges recounted whenever eldercare is mentioned, whether in a classroom, at a community gathering, on an airplane, or even in casual conversation.

I sensed a ripple of curiosity in the audience as I mentioned Viktor Frankl's logotherapy and its relevance to the issues of our times. As has been my experience nearly everywhere I've spoken over the years, this audience resonated with Frankl's three principle ways of finding meaning: doing a deed, loving, and even through suffering.

As we continued with an animated discussion of the relevance of finding meaning in today's world of uncertainty, a lanky young man seated in the back of the room stood and simply stated: "Dr. Marr Burdman, here in this audience is our very own poet, Marjorie Pizer, who has lots to say about meaning. I think her poem 'Web of the World' is spot on!"

As this young man motioned excitedly toward the front row, a slender, sandy-haired woman smiled demurely. Of course, I immediately invited her to speak! Marjorie Pizer graciously accepted and rose to recite her poem in one of the most confident and resonant voices I've ever heard:

Web of the World

In the whole web woven of the being of the world
Each of us has a place,
A small corner of the tapestry uniquely ours,
Spun in with our times and those around us.
We weave our own corner into its own shape

And all the tiny shapes become the whole,
And the whole moulds the little shapes
Until all are become part of one another.
No matter how small, all are required;
No matter how unimportant, all are necessary;
Each touches the whole and becomes a part of it.
Even you, even a small lizard, touches and changes
The skirts of the universe.

Silence engulfed the room! Pizer's poem struck a chord that provided a potent backdrop to the theme of the day. Later I learned that Marjorie Pizer was a friend of the prolific American poet, May Sarton, and that they corresponded regularly. May Sarton's words affirmed high regard for Ms. Pizer's poetry: "How rare the singular simplicity and depth of Marjorie Pizer's poems has become! Reading her I am given back a fresh way of experiencing myself. I am nourished."

Whether poet or philosopher, gerontology advocate or social activist, parent or grandparent, a basic and enduring human value is the ability to nourish oneself and others through recognizing our mutuality. Viktor Frankl taught me that the motivating force behind human behavior is the pursuit of meaning—a life-affirming search that propels us forward. In my global health work, I have observed his approach validated innumerable times by the "person in the street."

That inextinguishable search for purpose and meaning is a primary need for humans the world over. In whatever part of the world's web that we are experiencing at any given time, we're forced to ask ourselves: "What am I here for?" "What is my task?" "What is my assignment for this day?" "What's it all about?" "Why me?" "Why *not* me?"

Indeed, what kept Frankl alive through his horrendous trauma and personal losses in the concentration camps was his vision that, if he survived, he would share a critical message with the world. He would demonstrate that there are antidotes to despair. Though his writings were confiscated and destroyed by prison camp guards, he managed to reconstruct the essence of his work on bits and pieces of paper. When he was miraculously released, very near death, he redrafted his manuscript in nine days, and that eventually led to the publication of his classic book, *The Doctor and the Soul.*

Frankl's wisdom continues to reverberate globally and is especially pertinent to the critical questions: *Why is there so much despair? Why are we encountering so much pain in our midst and what can we do about it?*

Alienation—a sense of estrangement or abandonment, of not belonging—is characterized by loss of interest and lack of initiative, an inner emptiness.

Have you experienced feelings of "not belonging?" I sometimes hear clients and friends say "everything is so difficult; I feel as if I am on another planet." Indeed, what finally moves people to seek help is often this utterly painful feeling of disconnection.

People who seem to be most resilient and balanced are those who strive for a purpose worthy of their efforts. They are engaged in life. Yet, even the most upbeat individuals experience periodic episodes of "down time" when questions loom: "Am I just spinning my wheels?" "What is this all about?" "What am I here for?"

I sometimes hear people say, "Who would miss me if I didn't show up?" "Is it all worth it?" Have you ever asked yourself any of these questions? Life's meaning differs from person to person, from day to day, and even from hour to hour. What matters—what really matters—is the specific meaning we experience at any given moment. Indeed, the present moment is where we live!

Each of us has a personal vocation or mission that demands fulfillment. And each of our tasks is as unique as the specific opportunity to implement it. Yes, we all belong to that "web of the world!"

Yet, have you ever awakened with a sensation of dread? Ever had that feeling of not knowing how to begin to cope with the demands on your life? Have you ever felt like pulling the blankets over your head and just staying put?

You are not alone.

Sometimes it feels like we are surrounded by darkness and we doubt that we'll ever move beyond the gloom. Perhaps it is not the absence of despair that we seek. Rather, it may be that through the depths of despair we are able to come to a deeper understanding of our place in the wheel of life.

"Without darkness
nothing comes to birth,
as without light,
nothing flowers."

—MAY SARTON

"Be not afraid of life.
Believe that life is worth living,
and your belief
will help create the fact."

—WILLIAM JAMES

"If one has courage,
nothing can dim the light
that shines from within."

—MAYA ANGELOU

Reflections:

Three
Review the Stepping Stones
of Your Life

"We shall not cease from exploration
And the end of all our exploring
Will be to arrive where we started
And know the place for the first time."

—T. S. ELIOT

Life Review as a Pathway to Wholeness

As our myths of invulnerability give way and we recognize the transitory nature of life, we tend to become more introspective. I've been very interested in life review since the day I heard Robert Butler speak about its relationship to meaningful aging. Dr. Butler, geriatrician and Pulitzer-prize winning author of *Why Survive: Growing Old in America* visited the University of Washington in the autumn of 1978 shortly after taking the reins as the founding director of the National Institute on Aging. At the time, I was a new faculty member working with the Department of Health Education and the interdisciplinary Institute on Aging at the University of Washington.

Butler, a wise and compassionate man, spoke of life review as a basic human need—putting one's life in order and making sense of it in the process. He observed that many health care providers considered reminiscing to be a sign of senility and thus they stereotyped older people as living meaningless lives. In response to such negativity, he coined the term *ageism*.

Memories as Quarries of Recollections

I've learned that our memories are quarries of recollections that can be mined, allowing a renewed capacity for free association and a remarkable clarity of recaptured tastes, smells, and other sensations. Life review is a normal developmental process; recalling and reminiscing over past events can provide a unique opportunity for integrating the past and bridging across generations.

Means of evoking memory and facilitating life review that I find particularly effective are:

—*Written or taped autobiographies.* Telling our stories can be a vehicle to greater self-acceptance. Recording our thoughts and experiences may even allow recognition or acceptance of the "wisdom within."

—*Pilgrimages.* Most of us live some distance from our origins. Sometimes we have faint recollections of places of significance. A pilgrimage back to those sites can bring resolution or even unexpected fulfillment.

—*Reunions.* Related to the longing to revisit old places is the desire to "see one more time" family as well as persons with whom we grew up, went to school, or worked. Reunions provide an invaluable opportunity to reminisce and catch up on intervening events.

—*Genealogy.* As we age, we tend to become more curious about our forebears, as if half-expecting them to form a reception committee to orient us to our place in history. Genealogy research can provide a link to ancestors and to branches of the family tree. The advent of the study of the human genome has opened a whole new avenue to learn about ancestors that we could not have dreamed possible until very recently.

—*Memorabilia, scrapbooks, photo albums, old letters.* Probably the most accessible contact with the past for most of us is through our keepsakes and written or pictorial records.

—*Reflection on one's life work.* This is a challenging task that is probably more demanding than expected. We ask ourselves such questions as: "What have I contributed?" "Have I been authentic?" "What now?" "What next?"

When we share memories with an empathic listener, the overarching benefit is that the sharing itself can serve as a vehicle for acceptance of past events. Compassionate listening is acknowledging the significance of another's life experiences.

Listening is an Act of Love

A contemporary approach to life review is Story Corps, a project initiated by David Isay and National Public Radio (NPR). Isay described Story Corps in his 2007 book, *Listening is an Act of Love*: "Truly listening and giving your sincere attention to another can be a most therapeutic and loving activity."

Story Corps recordings, as heard on NPR and archived in the Library of Congress, have been inspiring people since 2003. In 2015, Isay was honored with the prestigious TED prize as well as a MacArthur "Genius Grant" in recognition of his work, which is taking this form of life review to a global level. David Isay encourages people everywhere, of all ages and circumstances, to join in. (To learn the locations of story booths across the USA, visit the URL www.storycorps.net.)

If a visit to a Story Corps booth is not convenient, Isay says "Do it yourself. Conduct your own interview and ask the questions you've always wanted to ask. You'll be surprised by the power of the experience." Wherever you are, whether with family or someone you just met, you can participate by voicing your own stories and listening to stories of those around you.

Start the process by figuring out whom you want to interview, whether a grandparent, an old friend, or your parents. Remind the storyteller that you think the story is important and that it will be valuable to future generations. Let that person know you would be pleased to hear and to record his or her story.

Some questions you may choose to ask are:

- What is the most important lesson you have learned in life?
- What are you most proud of?

- Do you have any regrets?
- What was the happiest moment of your life? The saddest?
- Is there something about yourself that you think no one knows?
- How would you like to be remembered?

Add your own questions or invite the person telling the story to add questions. It can be a rich and fulfilling reciprocal experience.

Generations Remember

Life review may also be considered a form of oral history. Recollections of historic events and the era in which they occurred are valuable eyewitness accounts of a nation's heritage. Tom Brokaw's 2004 book *The Greatest Generation* shows the value of gathering stories and experiences of those he called "extraordinary-ordinary" people. He aptly illustrates the power of recollection and the value of historical documentation.

On the heels of this book, Tom Brokaw wrote *Boom: Voices of the Sixties* (2007). When I heard him interviewed on NPR, I was struck by his comments about the period from 1963 to 1974 as "the '60s." He justified that definition by saying "history rarely cuts neatly by numbers." Then he noted that we moved swiftly from the grey flannel suits of the '50s to the turbulence of the '60s. He described the assassination of President Kennedy in 1963 as the beginning of our loss of innocence.

Who could deny that the assassination of Kennedy impacted us forever? Perhaps it was a loss of innocence that we could not even fathom. Who alive then cannot remember vividly where they were when the news broke?

I was walking through the Sucre, Bolivia town plaza returning to the household where I lived as a Peace Corps Volunteer. I heard the news over a loudspeaker: "El Presidente de los Estados Unidos fue matado en Dallas, Texas" (The President of the United States of America was killed in Dallas, Texas). My ears could hear the words blurted out over the speakers, but my mind could not comprehend them.

President Kennedy killed? This could not be true. I was part of the Peace Corps that President Kennedy had invited us to join just the year before. I ran the two blocks to the place I called home on Calle Audencia and entered my room just to the right of the fountain in the courtyard. I was dazed and panting. As I slowly removed my shoes, I looked up and saw Señora Elena, the owner of the house, weeping in the courtyard just outside my window. She had heard the announcement, too. She asked me to sit with her near the radio in her room to listen as the news was broadcast over and over. My Bolivian "mother" tenderly held my hand in hers.

Then groups of townspeople began coming to the door to express their condolences. Kennedy was revered in Sucre. The community members saw the Peace Corps as Kennedy's volunteers. They mourned with us. People dressed in black, and for several days, only somber music played over the loudspeakers in the plaza. There was no television in Bolivia in 1963, so we relied solely on the radio as those heart-wrenching days following the assassination unfolded. I had never seen such an outpouring of shock and grief. We were numbed by disbelief.

In Brokaw's book, I was especially interested to read what he had to say about the three years leading up to Kennedy's death and particularly about the Peace Corps. I was dismayed that Tom Brokaw skipped over those early days of the '60s when I and hundreds of other young people responded to Kennedy's call:

> "Ask not what your country can do for you…
> Ask what you can do for your country."

Those years as a Peace Corps Volunteer and later, as a Peace Corps staff member, opened pathways that I had not dreamed possible. How could anyone leave this out of a book on the '60s? And why did Brokaw only mention Peace Corps in one paragraph of one page? I realized from my reaction that I was personally immersed in my own life review!

Another Generation

An indelible defining moment for the generation of my parents was the news of an attack on our country. I vividly remember the stories they told of that infamous day in 1941—December 7—the attack on Pearl Harbor.

My parents, Aunt Janet, and Uncle John, who was home on leave from the Army, were playing a card game of pinochle. Suddenly, the announcement that Pearl Harbor had been attacked by Japan interrupted the radio program playing in the background. My parents remembered Uncle John's handsome ruddy face going bloodless as he heard the news. He knew he would be called to duty immediately.

It wasn't until 55 years after that day that I would hear directly from Aunt Janet what this announcement meant for her and Uncle John. While I sat at her side around the clock in her California home as hospice nurses attended in her final days, I realized that listening was the most loving thing I could do for her.

Aunt Janet recalled those early days in Minnesota, her husband's career path, and its impact on the family. She spoke of her emotions—the confusing mixture of pride, fear, and resentment— when John was sent on missions and she shouldered all the responsibilities at home, including caring for their young children and her elderly parents (my maternal grandparents).

Aunt Janet spoke with deep regret about having not achieved some of her goals. But she also spoke with pride about her civic accomplishments which included numerous awards and accolades. She told me about honors Uncle John had received that she found among his papers only after his death. John never mentioned them, or perhaps she had not been listening if he did! Then the floodgates opened as she spoke of all their missed opportunities for communication. I was reminded of a song by Mike Rutherford and B. A. Robertson (1988), "The Living Years":

> "It's too late when we die
> To admit we don't see eye to eye...
> I just wish I could have told him
> In the living years."

"Our happiness or unhappiness
depends far more
on the way we meet the events of life
than on
the nature of those events themselves."

—WILHELM VON HUMBOLT

"What lies behind us
and what lies before us
are tiny matters
compared to what lies
within us."

—RALPH WALDO EMERSON

"Be patient toward
all that is unsolved in your heart
and try to love the questions themselves."

—RAINER MARIA RILKE

Reflections:

Four
Accept Life's Transitions

"Come to the edge!"

        "We can't, we're afraid."

"Come to the edge!"

        "We can't, we will fall."

"Come to the edge!"

      And they came,
      He pushed them,
      And they flew.

        — GUILAUME APOLINAIRE

Edges… oh, edges! How many times have you been invited to the edge? How often have you felt yourself on the edge of a precipice? What happens? Fear at first—of course. We are all afraid.

That poem, "Come to the Edge," was read by the Swiss psychiatrist Dr. Elisabeth Kübler-Ross as more than 50 people of all walks of life—physicians, nurses, social workers, dying patients, bereaved daughters, sons, and parents—stood around a bonfire one crisp autumn evening at a Franciscan retreat center near Three Rivers, California in 1977. We had just concluded an intensive weeklong workshop titled "Life, Death, and Transitions." It was an invitation to face our fears of the unknown. Among the participants was a woman whose entire family—mother, father, and brother—had died in the preceding six months. She was numb with grief and nearly mute. And there was the midlife couple in deep grief over the death of their 18-year-old son, a high school valedictorian, bound for an Ivy League university. He died in a car crash after an all-night graduation party. That father's intense grief was expressed with raw fury; fury directed toward his son for having attended the party and anger at himself for letting his only son go that fateful night.

There was the emergency room physician whose younger brother had been murdered in a drive-by shooting, furious that the police had botched the investigation. He never learned who had killed his brother and he vowed revenge. Other attendees at the gathering were grieving losses of all kinds: death, lost love, purposelessness, meaninglessness. Many expressed feelings of deep despair—not knowing how to grasp the fraying fabric of their lives.

Rita Ward, a midlife widow, traveled from her home in Australia after Jack, her beloved husband and soulmate, had died. Bereft after her abrupt loss, she felt totally unprepared to raise their two young boys. So intense was the outpouring of community grief that Rita's neighbors collected funds for her to make the trip. They had heard of the groundbreaking work of Dr. Kübler-Ross and thought Rita could benefit from the trip. Indeed, she did. Shortly thereafter, she became the organizer for Elisabeth's work throughout Australia and to this day is a respected advocate for palliative care.

Lifelong friendships were forged through Elisabeth's commitment to opening communication lines among participants. Rita has become one of my dearest friends. Over the years, she has facilitated my work and introductions to leaders in both Australia and New Zealand, resulting in invitations for me to present workshops and seminars in both countries on our universal search for meaning throughout the lifespan. In Australia as well as in New Zealand I've had extraordinary teaching and learning experiences. My decades-long collaboration with Joy Nugent, a palliative care nursing leader and founder of Nurselink in Australia has greatly expanded my awareness of the multifaceted aspects of end-of-life care and the vital importance of teamwork and communication among health care providers and families (see the URL www. nurselinkfoundation.com).

A hallmark of all Kübler-Ross workshops was the mix of participants and their experiences. Yes, she wanted to reach health care providers, clergy, funeral directors, and other professionals. But even more, she sought to reach out to the dying and the bereaved. Elisabeth's primary motivation was to teach us all about letting go of fear! Indeed, during the intensely emotional week we learned from one another and acknowledged our common vulnerability along with our common humanity. I could not have predicted the interconnectivity that would manifest from that experiential week of learning and grieving and healing.

In the most amazing and perceptive way, Elisabeth guided each of us throughout that week to peel away our layers of resistance to face our own issues and pain, much like peeling away an onion layer by layer. She knew precisely when to allow silence and quiet compassion to do the teaching as we shared our stories one by one in a safe and nurturing atmosphere among the pines of northern California.

At that time, I was teaching at the University of Oregon and eager to take back extracurricular content for my gerontology students. Little did I know what a phenomenal experience it would be, a week of intensive learning that no textbook could come close to offering.

Throughout the workshop, Elisabeth shared numerous examples of how we treat life's grief and pain as something to be avoided at all costs. But, she asserted, "These experiences are really gifts." Then she spoke of the "little deaths," the losses that occur in all our lives: loss of physical capacities, friends, jobs, security, stature, homes, and others.

What about the "gift" of pain and loss? That was a big one to swallow. But then I remembered those three ways of finding meaning: through love, through service, and even through suffering. When I mentioned my commitment to integrating Frankl's philosophy and psychology into my own work, Elisabeth responded: "Yes, Geri, when any of us look back at the anguish, suffering, and traumas in our lives, we will see that these are periods of immense growth."

> "It is only when we truly know and understand
> that we have a limited time on earth—
> and that we have no way of knowing
> when our time is up—
> that we begin to live each day to the fullest,
> as if it were the only one we had."
>
> —ELISABETH KÜBLER-ROSS

Dr Kübler-Ross' pioneering work impacted people around the globe and opened conversations about end-of-life care that were extraordinary at the time. Now, some four decades later, there is more openness surrounding the subject of death and dying, but the process is still shrouded in fear. A current best-selling book, *Being Mortal* by Dr. Atul Gawande (2014), is addressing this fear directly and re-energizing a crucial conversation among health care providers and consumers alike. Among other contemporary authors covering the subject are highly respected researchers and practitioners Drs. Ira Byock and George Bonanno, both of whom interpret their extensive research related to end-of-life care as well as bereavement and life after loss. Joy Nugent's 2015 book, *As Good as Good-Byes Get: A Window into Death and Dying* highlights the essential role of teamwork and compassion in health care.

I am often reminded to pay close attention to events that have guided me thus far and to recognize teachable moments as well as the teachers appearing on my path today. Lessons learned from those who lit the fires for my growth continue to be an integral part of my life. And I revisit and ruminate on subtle lessons that present themselves. Facing our fears of the unknown and recognizing humanity's interconnections are recurring themes that I believe are especially relevant in today's world of uncertainty.

Perspective on the Hopi Message

In workshops I present in Arizona, I've invited LouVina Majo, a wise and compassionate woman who lives between the worlds of her Hopi Nation and Prescott, where she counsels and teaches about Native American traditions. LouVina shares valuable insights into the spiritual nature of Hopi culture and its ancient life ways as expressed in a complex interweaving of ceremony, stories, songs, art, and agriculture. She underscores the importance of sharing stories for generations to come.

In her clear, confident voice, LouVina reads an urgent message from her Hopi Elders that is making its way around the world. The Elders of Oraibi, Arizona, implore us to ponder the great questions and to seek meaningful paths:

> You have been telling the people that this is the eleventh hour.
> Now you must go back and tell the people that this is The Hour.
> Here are the things that must be considered:
> Where are you living?
> What are you doing?

What are your relationships?

Are you in right relation?

Where is your water?

Know your garden.

It is time to speak your Truth.

Create your community.

Be good to each other.

And do not look outside yourself for the leader.

This could be a good time!

There is a river flowing now very fast.

It is so great and swift that there are those who will be afraid.

They will try to hold on to the shore.

They will feel like they are being torn apart, and they will suffer greatly.

Know the river has its destination.

The elders say we must let go of the shore, push off toward the middle of the river.

Keep our eyes open, and our heads above the water.

See who is there with you and celebrate.

At this time in history, we are to take nothing personally, least of all ourselves!

For the moment we do, our spiritual growth and journey comes to a halt.

The time of the lone wolf is over.

Gather yourselves!

Banish the word "struggle" from your attitude and vocabulary.

All that we do now must be done in a sacred manner and in celebration.

We are the Ones we have been waiting for.

"This we know, the earth does not
belong to us, we belong to the earth.
This we know, all things are connected,
like the blood which unites one family.
All things are connected."

—CHIEF SEATTLE

"We all need to tell our story
and to understand our story....
We need for life to signify,
to touch the eternal,
to understand the mysterious
and to find out who we are."

—JOSEPH CAMPBELL

"Live each day
as if
your life had just begun."

—JOHANN WOLFGANG VON GOETHE

Reflections:

Five
Discover Your Path with Heart

"Your vision becomes clearer
when you look inside your heart.
Who looks outside, dreams.
Who looks inside, awakens."

—CARL JUNG

Just what is a path with heart? When we ask ourselves whether we are following a path with heart, we discover that no one else can define what our path should be. Where do we put our time, our energy, and our commitment? When we let the questions themselves penetrate our being, the answers often arise. It is a unique opportunity to open to the spiritual nature of life itself.

When we allow ourselves to be still and to listen deeply, even for a few seconds, we can learn the extent to which we are responding to our own path. Silence speaks! Listening within is the key to understanding in every circumstance. It is an essential ingredient, a vital part of a pathway to authenticity and purposefulness.

Success and Happiness as By-Products

I believe that we all seek meaning regardless of circumstances; a path with heart is in reality one that is worthy of our efforts! Many spiritual traditions teach that fulfillment and peace of mind come from making the most of our unique gifts and abilities, from "giving" rather than "getting."

The propensity to seek pleasure—and power—is increasingly visible in our world today. Yet people are often plagued by a feeling of vagueness, an inner emptiness. Viktor Frankl maintained that success and happiness come as by-products, never to be pursued for the sake of acquisition or aggrandizement.

Martin Luther King, Jr. similarly said:

> We are prone to judge success by the index of our salaries or the size of our automobiles rather than by the quality of our service and relationship to humanity.... Everyone must decide whether he will walk in the light of creative altruism or in the darkness of destructive selfishness. Life's most urgent question is, what are you doing for others?

You Only Have What You Give

Chilean best-selling author Isabel Allende spoke at a luncheon I attended in Seattle a few years after her beloved 28-year-old daughter, Paula, died in her arms. During that first year of deep grief, everything stopped for her: "However, that year also gave me an opportunity to reflect upon my journey and the principles that hold me together. I discovered that there is consistency in my beliefs, my writing, and the way I lead my life." She added, "Paula taught me a lesson that is now my mantra: 'You only have what you give. It's by spending yourself that you become rich.'"

Stand Tall with Deep Roots

"Walking the World in a Sacred Way" was the theme of a conference led by anthropologist Angeles Arrien among the majestic Red Rocks of Sedona, Arizona. I distinctly remember the moment Arrien bid us to "Stand tall—with deep roots—and know who you are!"

That invitation resonated with me, a reminder of Albert Einstein's words that I had just read on a park bench plaque: "Look deep into nature, and there you will understand everything better."

Trees are at once a symbol of growth, renewal, and transformation. I see the miraculous renewing capacity of the tree, ever changing with the seasons, as a metaphor for the process of human life in its continuous growth and unfoldment. And the symbolism of the evergreen tree with its stately branches is life itself deeply rooted and connected to its source.

In Eugene, Oregon, which I call my "Heart Home," I was fortunate to live in a thickly forested area when I taught gerontology and community health education courses at the University of Oregon in the mid-1970s. Each morning a local radio station played "Annie's Song" by John Denver—"You wake up my senses/Like a night in the forest." That song was a magnificent reminder to awaken to a new day with all its challenges and opportunities for growth.

My memories of a gnarled old oak tree and the white-tailed deer that came to lick a salt block we had placed at the foot of that particular tree are as vivid now as they were several decades ago.

Why?

Trees have a personal emotional significance for me and for many people I meet along my path. In fact, I find that most people have deep feelings and associations connected with trees. In my workshops and seminars, I frequently invite participants to remember a tree that was significant in their lives. Then we share stories… "once upon a time…." The stored memories that come pouring fourth are breathtaking.

At a workshop in Seattle, Mark, an outdoor enthusiast, recalled his reaction of "total awe" the first time he passed through the magnificent giant sequoia trees in Northern California, home to the most massive trees on this planet. Mark is an avid proponent of the Sierra Club and noted with sadness that over half of the remaining sequoia groves are at risk. He asked us to join in the effort to protect the Giant Sequoia National Monument. He said "we need to work for protection of these majestic trees—these living monuments." With a quivering voice, Mark went on to say that "without permanent protection, even trees that take two centuries or more to grow are at risk."

I think Mark is among those people who have such vivid memories of trees, as well as the events and emotions of those recollections, that the idea of communication with trees seems quite natural. Trees evoke strength and protection.

Viktor Frankl was fond of relating a story of his encounter with a terminally ill girl who knew she was dying. Asked how she could be so cheerful even though her time was short, his young patient pointed to a small tree just outside her window. She said: "I am able to talk with the tree; it is a friend." Frankl asked if the tree replied to her. She answered: "Yes, it says: 'I am here, I am here, I am Life.'"

Standing Tall

Viktor Frankl, though slight in physical stature, stood tall. His exhortation: "Listen to the person in the street; he or she may be your teacher!" came to me recently as I stopped by the extensive and ever-expanding—and expensive—Bellevue Square shopping mall, just east of Seattle.

Bellevue is a community of affluence and rapid growth. Bell Square (as it is called by locals) is just a couple of miles from Bill and Melinda Gates' neighborhood. I point to this geographical fact because, as among the wealthiest people on the planet, Bill and Melinda Gates and their Foundation have a commitment to global health and well-being that is unrivaled in its philanthropic mission. In the United States, their work seeks to ensure that all people—especially those with the fewest resources—have access to opportunities they need to succeed in school and life. Their global mission is based on the belief that "everyone deserves the chance to live a healthy, productive life."

Communities of Complex and Challenging Lives

In Bellevue, however, there is another, less visible, community just a couple of miles to the east of Bell Square: a community of relatively recent immigrants from all parts of the globe. It is a community of people with complex and challenging lives that has caught the attention of the affluent, including the owner of Bell Square. Tucked in among the elegant shops is the LifeSpring Thrift Shop. A cadre of volunteers maintains a space filled with used clothing, toys, books, and sundry other items donated by area residents as they enter the mall to shop at Nordstroms, Tiffany, Coach, Ann Taylor, and other upscale stores.

I like to drop by the thrift shop because there are incredible bargains to be had—some slightly worn and some never-worn garments from the likes of Eileen Fisher, Dana Buchman, Kate Spade, and other "names"—you get the picture. Also, there are lessons to be learned!

Quiet Grace

The search for significance has many faces, and the humblest among us are often the greatest teachers. Late one afternoon, as I looked around the LifeSpring Thrift Shop, a tall East African woman with a tiny babe in arms walked up to me and held a fuchsia-colored raw silk dress next to her high-cheek-boned ebony face. She asked, "Would I dare wear this?"

I answered: "Of course; it is beautiful!" I commented that her baby was precious; she smiled and went about looking through the racks of children's clothing. Then I overheard this humble yet regal woman quietly speak to a child in the yellow alcove filled with used toys: "Now place them all back on the shelves," she said, ever so gently.

I looked into the toy-lined niche and saw a bright-eyed boy about three years old playing with a John Deere tractor on the floor. I said, "Oh, you have another child!" She smiled at me and said "two more," just as a kindergarten-age girl with pink ribbons in her tightly braided hair peeked up from the Disney puzzle she was piecing together.

The mother-child bond was palpable. I commented, "Your children are so well mannered and you are very patient and kind." She looked at me with the most gracious smile and softly whispered, "I love them so."

As this mother paid for her few articles of clothing and left the store with her three children in tow, I suddenly realized that I had encountered a teacher. That mother touched my life with her quiet grace. Though I do not know her name, I remember her often. She stands tall… with deep roots!

"Do not go where the path may lead, go
instead where there is no path
and leave a trail."

RALPH WALDO EMERSON

"To live means sharing one another's
space, dreams, sorrows;
contributing our ears to hear,
our eyes to see,
our arms to hold,
our hearts to love."

—PAUL TILLICH

"Hope is the thing with feathers
that perches in the soul
and sings the tune without words
and never stops at all."

EMILY DICKENSON

Reflections:

Six
Release the
Burden of Resentments

"Forgiveness is a choice that we make
to release our past and heal our present."

—FREDRICK LUSKIN

What allowed Viktor Frankl to move through the world with his message of purpose in every day and every experience? How did he and countless others manage to forgive the unforgivable? How have innocent victims of violence and injustice managed to move on with newfound purpose and passion?

I am struck by the perseverance and courage of former US Congresswoman Gabby Giffords and her astronaut husband, Mark Kelly, as they have responded to the tragic mass shooting in Tucson, Arizona that changed their lives forever. They have transformed their energies into a purpose that they could not have imagined just a few short years ago.

In a recent letter requesting support for their current work on gun control, Mark writes:

> On January 8, 2011 there was no countdown clock.
>
> That phone call from a staffer for my wife sent me hurtling on a path with no clear trajectory. He said a man walked up to Gabby at an event she was holding for constituents in Tucson, shot her at point-blank range, and she fell to the ground. She was the shooter's first victim. He fired 30 shots randomly into the line of people gathered to talk to Gabby. Police said every one of his bullets pierced a human being. In 15 seconds, he emptied his magazine. It contained 33 bullets and there were 33 victims.
>
> In the long, hard months since then, Gabby, who was shot cleanly all the way through her brain—in the front and out the back—has slowly and step by relentless and strenuous step recovered one small capacity at a time.
>
> The words she once struggled to speak so meticulously one at a time, have turned into sentences. She now walks without a cane.
>
> And our new path? It has a clear trajectory...
>
> We want to prevent what happened to Gabby and others including those precious children who were killed in the school in Newtown, Connecticut... from happening to others.
>
> We all need the courage... the will to do it.
>
> We must stop America's epidemic of gun violence.

Gabby wrote:

> The time is now... time to be bold and courageous.
>
> As Mark reminds me, I used to talk before the shooting about how blessed we were... an astronaut and a congresswoman, newlyweds, profoundly in love, trying to start a family, a limitless future before us... Today we are challenged to make a difference.
>
> Words are difficult for me now. But there is one I can speak with clarity and conviction—that word is ENOUGH!

Forgiveness is at the Heart of Healing

In today's world, the very idea of forgiveness is repugnant to many who live by "an eye for an eye and a tooth for a tooth." Gandhi is said to have countered these words with: "If we live by an eye for an eye and a tooth for a tooth... soon we will all be blind and toothless."

Have we been blinded by our urge to get even? What allows some people to let go while others only grow embittered?

I have known individuals whose resentments have virtually destroyed their lives. And I've known others who pushed through painful experiences to a new sense of purpose. What is the vehicle that permits such a breakthrough for some?

One of my dearest friends, Louise, and her husband were returning home from a dinner celebrating her birthday some years ago when a drunken driver careened across the I-90 bridge between Seattle and Mercer Island, Washington, hitting their car head on. Paramedics were on the scene within minutes and Louise was rushed by ambulance to Harborview, a world-class trauma center in Seattle. She was placed on life support for several days before she died of severe head injuries.

I immediately headed to Harborview when I received that shattering call from her husband, Dave, telling me that Louise was probably "brain dead." To this day, I vividly recall the sight of my precious friend bound in bandages and hooked up to numerous tubes with intensive care machinery beeping relentlessly. Louise's husband paced the hallway, consumed with rage. Rage at the young man who was driving while intoxicated and who escaped injury in the accident. Dave's thoughts were of revenge and, in his grief, he spoke of nothing else—"I'll get back at that guy who maimed Louise!"

After months of deep grief and profuse anger, Dave had a remarkable change of heart and attitude. What prompted it? He could not explain except to say, "Louise held a light that kept me from stumbling. Now I need to hold that light." Dave immersed himself in community work with Mothers Against Drunk Driving. He set about volunteering with community education campaigns and helping others deal with their grief. Though his pain from the loss of his beloved Louise is inestimable, through service to others he was liberated from the unrelenting angst of unforgiveness.

Forgiveness has many faces. When I heard Azim Khamisa speak of his 20-year-old son, Tariq, murdered by a 14-year-old gang-member recruit in Southern California, I was astounded by yet another account of tragedy turned into a powerful commitment to service. Azim Khamisa's dedication in remembrance of his young son touched me deeply.

Mr. Khamisa, a dignified and articulate man, shares his commitment with individuals and groups throughout the USA. I heard him speak of his newfound life purpose at a Peace Alliance meeting in Washington, D.C. He recalled the shock and intensity of his grief and that of Tariq's mother when they heard the news. Azim said the heart-wrenching shriek on the other end of the phone line when he called Tariq's mother is forever embedded in his memory.

But Azim was astonished by his own response. Even in the midst of intense grief, he had no interest in demanding revenge or retribution; instead, he saw two of Americas' sons lost—one to death and one to the state prison system: "From the outset, I saw victims on both ends of the gun.

I will mourn Tariq's death for the rest of my life. Now, however, my grief has been transformed into a powerful commitment to change. Change is urgently needed in a society where children kill children."

All of us can read lofty words of forgiveness and repeat them. But to live the lessons is quite another story. Certainly, I remember many times when I felt it impossible to let go of resentments. And I ruminated over the actions, reactions, and even inactions of others that led to those burdensome feelings. But over the years in my personal search for meaning, I have come to recognize that, difficult as it may seem, forgiveness is at the heart of healing.

Wise teachers along the way have reminded me that forgiveness releases the baggage of the past and lifts the burdens of resentment and remorse. When we are mentally free of these emotions, we are more prone to activate our heart of compassion.

A Sure Remedy

While going through papers and sundry items left by my mother when she passed away, I came across a writing on which the words *"very important!"* appeared.

"A Sure Remedy" by Charles Fillmore gives a prescription for forgiveness:

Sit each evening and mentally forgive everyone against whom you have any ill will or antipathy. If you fear or if you are prejudiced against even an animal, mentally ask forgiveness of it and send it thoughts of love. If you have accused anyone of injustice, if you have discussed anyone unkindly, if you have criticized or gossiped about anyone, withdraw your words by asking in silence for forgiveness.

If you have had a falling out with friends or relatives, see all things and all persons as they really are—pure spirit—and send them your strongest thoughts of love. Be patient, loving, and kind under all circumstances.

Forgiveness allows some extraordinary people to turn the burden of pain from their profound losses into calls for action. Gabby Giffords and her husband Mark Kelly work tirelessly on ending gun violence. Louise's husband Dave released some of his angst by volunteering with Mothers Against Drunk Driving. Azim Khamisa uses the memory of his beloved son to raise awareness of the urgent need to end the senseless killing of children.

Longstanding resentments, regardless of their origin, imprison us; forgiveness can provide a reset button inviting the possibility to live more purposefully.

"Forgiveness does not change the past,
but it does enlarge the future."

—PAUL BOESE

"To forgive
is to set a prisoner free
and to discover
the prisoner was you."

—LEWIS SMEDES

"Let every step I take
be one of forgiveness."

—GERALD JAMPOLSKY

"The practice of forgiveness
is our most important contribution
to the healing of the world."

—MARIANNE WILLIAMSON

Reflections:

Seven
Embrace Your Age

> "Old age, to the unlearned, is winter;
> to the learned, it is harvest time."
>
> YIDDISH PROVERB

I am frequently inundated with notices about "anti-aging" books, conferences, workshops, potions, formulas, and sundry other promotions to counteract the "problems of aging." I invariably react with "why anti-aging?" as I press the delete key or toss flyers into the recycling basket beneath my desk.

That ubiquitous term "anti-aging" has crept into our common language, adding to the negative perceptions surrounding the process of maturing and developing across the lifespan. Stereotypes contribute to the overwhelming challenges encountered among many older adults today; loneliness, loss of self-esteem, and feelings of hopelessness are rampant. Of course, these are not confined to older persons; the experience of despair occurs among people of all ages when a sense of purpose and meaning is waning.

Now, don't get me wrong! I definitely believe self-care is integral to enhancing the quality of our lives, day by day. Recognizing the interrelationship of body, mind, and spirit is critical to achieving a state of wellness and optimal functioning at any age. And, of course, ever-emerging research findings concerning health across the lifespan are bringing vital information to the forefront, but why not call this pursuit something other than "anti-aging?" How about "living into fullness?" Or "redefining calendar years?" Or simply "maturing healthfully?"

Enhancing quality of life regardless of age, gender, or social circumstances is at the heart of my work. And I do not call the incremental process of growth and development across the lifespan anything but aging or maturing.

Shape-Shifting Events Changing Perceptions

Over the years, many seminal events have contributed to my perspectives on aging, yet none compare with that first meeting with Viktor Frankl in Puerto Rico in the late 1960s; it was a pivotal time in my personal and professional development. The last time I had the privilege of learning directly from Dr. Frankl was in the springtime of 1989, when he addressed the American Society on Aging in Washington, D.C. Then in his 80s, slightly bent with a shock of white hair and a slower gait as well as diminishing eyesight, Dr. Frankl took to the lectern with his characteristic powerful voice and strength of conviction. He repeated his timeless message of unconditional meaningfulness throughout the lifespan, imploring attendees to visualize new images of aging. I came away from that conference keenly attuned to the growing awareness that a search for meaning is innate to human beings regardless of age. It's a deep longing for a purposeful path.

Gerontologists, clergy, and academics, as well as health and social service providers, were all gathered at that national event. Frankl's unwavering message of the vital importance of discovery throughout all phases of life sparked my interest in exploring new dimensions of aging.

It was my last opportunity to converse directly with Drs. Viktor and Elly Frankl, and to express my heartfelt gratitude to each of them for their extraordinary work that fuels my passion for helping people seek purpose and meaning throughout the lifespan. Elly Frankl is often called "the light that accompanied the messenger." I still hear from colleagues and former students who also were deeply moved by the radiant presence of this remarkable couple who, for decades, shared their life and love with the world. The Frankls' message of unconditional meaningfulness was a wake-up call to gerontologists. I believe it served as a precursor to what is now called the *conscious aging movement*.

At about that same time, the groundbreaking work of Harvard psychologist Ellen Langer was being recognized. The central question of her research focused on whether one's mental attitude can reverse effects of aging. In studies spanning more than a quarter century, Langer showed that mental attitude can indeed reverse some effects of aging and can also contribute to improving physical health.

Langer's unconventional studies have long suggested what brain science is now revealing: Our experiences are formed by the words and ideas we attach to them. Langer is considered one of the early pioneers—along with figures like Jon Kabat-Zinn and Herbert Benson—whose work reveals a linkage between attitude and quality of life impacting vitality, energy, and overall well-being.

Conscious Aging

What then is conscious aging? Valuing each day as an opportunity for growth is at its very heart. It's also about expanding awareness of the potential for discovering meaning throughout the lifespan.

Just a few years after Frankl's challenge to the gerontological community, I participated in the first Conscious Aging conference in New York City sponsored by the Omega Institute, a holistic education center at the forefront of personal and professional development in areas ranging from health and psychology to multicultural arts and spirituality. Omega is renowned for its broad-based curriculum and unique community spirit; this 1992 gathering was the Institute's first journey into the field of gerontology. It was a transformative event with attendees responding to a call to explore "Conscious Aging: A Creative and Spiritual Journey."

At the outset, the conference organizers proposed a departure from the prevailing narrow view of aging as a clinical problem. Central to the discussions was the notion that to age consciously is to recognize that in every phase of our human journey we are changing, growing, and yes—aging.

Shining a courageous light on the full spectrum of the aging process proved to be a rallying point. A vibrant energy reverberated throughout the three-day conference as we discussed our understanding of aging, embracing the creative possibilities of celebrating maturity, honoring elders, mentoring, and integrating significance into every stage of our lives. Omega carried my book, *Joyful Aging*, in their conference bookstore. It was a unique opportunity to exchange impressions as we contemplated our visions for conscious aging. Of course, I shared my enthusiasm about Viktor Frankl's work and an emerging theme of our times: Discovering portals to significance throughout our lifespan.

Among the presenters whose extraordinary works continue to impact perceptions and attitudes about aging were the late Rabbi Zalman Schacter-Shalomi, founder of Sage-ing International (which can be found at the URL www.sage-ing.org); Harry (Rick) Moody, gerontologist and former academic director at the American Association of Retired Persons (AARP); and cultural anthropologist Mary Catherine Bateson.

Rabbi Schacter-Shalomi invited us to move into a new arena for appreciating the wisdom of age: "we must all pass through a gate of transformation that enables us to use our life experience to enrich our elder years, face mortality, repair relationships, and transmit wisdom to future generations." He reminded us that, among traditional cultures, older adults are seen as a source of knowledge, healing, and power. Indeed, elders are often the backbone of their community—the healers and the vision keepers.

Rick Moody posited: "Like multiple mirrors reflecting a single light, the variety of images, teachings, and mythologies from the Western psychological and Eastern mystical perspectives show us that growing old is an experience both personal and universal." Moody continues to have his finger on the pulse of gerontological matters. Among his multiple contributions to the field is the monthly "Human Values in Aging" electronic newsletter that highlights literature, conferences, and other current learning opportunities. Rick Moody's commitment to conscious aging continues unabated!

Mary Catherine Bateson presented a riveting perspective: "Life is an improvisational art form, and the interruptions, conflicted priorities, and demands that are part of all our lives can be seen as a source of wisdom. Living longer and under rapidly changing circumstances, we must improvise much of our lives."

Dr. Bateson's insightful perception of aging as an evolving art form leads me to frequently ponder the relevance of these words attributed to her anthropologist mother:

> "Never doubt that a small group of thoughtful, committed citizens can change the world. Indeed, it's the only thing that ever has."
>
> —MARGARET MEAD

Change and Challenge: Conscious Aging Today

Indeed, there is change afoot! And, of course, challenges abound. Yet the ripples from that 1992 Conscious Aging event in New York are visible and palpable today. Fast forward to the year 2015 and we find "conscious aging" entering our common lexicon and even being studied and discussed in academic as well as other professional circles. A couple of 2015 events that underscored the shift in consciousness include Seattle University's Search for Meaning Book Festival (see the URL www.seattleu.edu/searchformeaning) and the Transforming Aging Summit (found at the URL www.theshiftnetwork.com).

The Search for Meaning Book Festival, one of Seattle's largest literary events, brought 55 regional, national, and international authors who presented a range of ecumenical and secular perspectives on a quest for meaning across the lifespan. With well over 1000 participants from all walks of life, the event demonstrated the intense interest in this critical theme of our times. I was honored to be invited to present a workshop based on my book *Search for Significance: Finding Meaning in Times of Change, Challenge, and Chaos.*

The Transforming Aging Summit, a groundbreaking online series, was designed by the Shift Network to introduce people of all ages to conscious and positive aging. Its multidimensional perspective focused on the potential for purpose and continual growth throughout the lifespan. During this series, 18 leaders with diverse perspectives on positive aging were interviewed by Ron Pevny, Director of the Center for Conscious Eldering.

Some of the interviewees referred to that first Omega aging event in 1992 as the initiation that jump-started their personal commitments to conscious aging. Academicians Rick Moody and Robert Atchley spoke specifically about the contributions of Rabbi Zalman Schacter-Shalomi and his impact on their lives.

Richard Leider, author and proponent of purposeful living, mentioned his first encounter with Viktor Frankl. It seems that he stumbled upon an announcement in a hallway in

California that led him to meet and study with Dr. Frankl in San Diego years ago. Leider's fortuitous encounter with this great teacher brought back memories of my first meeting with Dr. Frankl at the University of Puerto Rico.

Richard Leider emphasized that aging well is about much more than improving physical health, mental acuity, and longevity; it is also essential to include purposeful growth throughout the lifespan.

While aging does come with its share of losses and diminishments, the multidimensional vision highlighted in The Transforming Aging series demonstrated that this process can also include vast possibilities for true fulfillment and growth in whatever circumstances we find ourselves. The speakers laid out expansive possibilities for the gifts elders can contribute to the world with the wisdom of decades of life experiences.

"To unfold one's truth within oneself
is the lifelong aspiration
of every human."

—RABINDRANATH TAGORE

"Winter is on my head,
but eternal Spring is in my heart."

—VICTOR HUGO

"It is age that teaches us to enjoy life,
to savor every moment of it,
to spend our time on what counts,
to be present where we are
and see it for the first time."

—JOAN CHITTISTER

Reflections:

Eight
Live Your Legacy

"When we cast our bread upon the waters,
we can presume that someone downstream
whose face we may never see
will benefit from our action."

—MAYA ANGELOU

We are shaped by what we think and what we do and how we regard the generative nature of life itself. A concern for guiding future generations is a hallmark of generativity, a term coined by Erik and Joan Erikson. Our legacy lies with the demonstration of our core values, our truths, and our care for others.

A superb example of *generativity in action* is Rachel Carson, author of *Silent Spring*; her legacy continues to significantly impact our lives. Through her works and deeds, Carson made a lasting contribution to the environmental movement. Born in the Allegheny valley town of Springdale, Pennsylvania, Carson's mother instilled in her a strong sense of independence and a love of nature. Carson held an ecological view of nature. She addressed the interconnectedness of all living things: humans, plants, animals, and farms as elements in the "web of life." *Silent Spring*, written in 1962, made her one of the most important authors of our time. Her plea and her legacy resonate loudly today:

"It's always so easy to assume that someone else is taking care of things. Trusting so-called authority is not enough. A sense of personal responsibility is what we desperately need."

Let Retrospectives Make Their Peace in Your Heart

Generativity is also reflected as a deep desire in parents' hearts to see their children realize their potential. As parents and grandparents, what we teach children is often what we must continue to learn ourselves. Finding one's purpose and *living it* reveals the significance of life itself. This discovery is an ongoing process that unfolds throughout the lifespan.

Years ago, when my friend and neighbor, Ann Gartrell, was approaching her transition from this earth plane, she wrote poetic notes to friends and family. Among her words,

these continue to touch me deeply:
"In the autumn of my life, let every leaf be shining gold;
Let retrospectives make their peace in my heart."

Kind-hearted, diminutive Ann was my neighbor and the mother of two young boys—they were my two sons' best friends. Though Ann was only in her late 30s when she passed, she demonstrated courage and maturity well beyond her years. Her constant reminder to her sons and their friends was to "live life now." When her strength waned in the final months of life, she consciously chose to use her precious remaining energy to explore the thickly wooded ravine near our home with the four young children in tow.

Ann recognized the importance of sharing her stories and insights with the young ones. All other obligations and chores fell to the bottom of her priority list. To this day, more than 30 years later, my sons remember Ann's stories of friendship and of the joys of nature, and her admonition to "live life purposefully." Through her gentle presence and reminiscing, Ann imparted important lessons to the young ones. She shared from the deep desire of every parent's heart to see children become who they are meant to be. Through sharing her personal stories, she taught them that there is a purpose and a catalyst for growth through every event, action, and deed.

Becoming Real

Do you remember *The Velveteen Rabbit*, a children's classic written in 1922 by Margery Williams? The heart of the story is the mystical and transformative power of love.

My maternal grandmother often recounted tales that reflected her own generative nature. Here is my recollection of that Velveteen rabbit story—as told to me by Grandma Annie Knowlton:

> For a long time, a certain stuffed bunny remained just a plaything in a child's nursery. But the bunny really didn't mind because he was able to carry on long philosophical discussions with an old skin horse who was very wise. It seems that one of the rabbit's favorite topics of conversation was about becoming Real. The skin horse patiently explained to the bunny that "Real is not how you are made. It's a thing that happens to you. It doesn't happen all at once… you become… it takes a long time. When a child loves you for a long time, not just to play with but really loves you, then you become Real."

Like the velveteen rabbit, I believe that we all long to become Real. Authenticity comes through living with commitment and purpose.

My Grandma Annie taught valuable lessons with her storytelling as well as through her exemplary deeds. She embroidered her favorite maxim on pillow slips that were handed down from my mother to me:

"Let every waking hour bring a lesson on its wing."

I've framed one of those embroidered pieces for each of my three beloved grandchildren—Chaison, Robert, and Malia, who reside in Kailua-Kona, Hawaii. They are my teachers, too! They gave me an experience that profoundly touched my heart:

I was relaxing on a lanai overlooking the majestic Pacific Ocean in Kailua-Kona with my Hawaiian family—my son Robert and his lovely wife Kalei along with other members of the *'ohana* (family) including about a dozen children ranging from two months to twelve years old. Suddenly Chaison, then about six years of age, interrupted his game of tag and rushed up to me shrieking, "Grandma Geri, what are those green lines on your hands?"

I quickly looked down, as I had never noticed any green lines on my hands! Chaison's urgency told me that he thought the backs of my hands posed an immediate health crisis. I was at once amused and speechless as Chaison anxiously pointed to the veins on the backs of my pale hands. An immediate hush came over the conversation as my son patiently explained to Chaison that there was no cause for alarm. "Grandma Geri is fine—when many people get older, the skin gets a bit thinner and sometimes their veins show through a little. Veins carry our blood around our bodies." Chaison, obviously relieved that no emergency measures were needed, shouted "Okay!" and dashed off to play with his cousins.

The adult conversation resumed, but after about 10 minutes, Chaison reappeared, pulling a canvas folding chair over beside me. Gently he took my right hand and ran his index finger up and down the back of my hand—tracing the veins. He said, ever so softly, "Grandma Geri, you might be a little bit old out here." Then as he clutched both his hands to his heart, he said, "but you are young in here!"

What precious gifts are grandchildren! I carry photos of them: Chaison, Robert James, and Malia Joy. Like grandmothers everywhere, I share their stories with anyone interested (as well as with those who politely indulge me)!

Recently, on an airplane a fellow traveler—another grandmother— said, "Oh yes, they open a chamber of your heart that you didn't even know existed!"

Among my favorite photos is one of Chaison dressed for a traditional *hula* celebration. He wears a *lei* fashioned from nuts of the kukui or candlenut tree (Aleurites moluccana). In ancient Hawaii, the oil-filled nuts of the kukui were used as lights, and Hawaii's native people look upon the tree as a symbol of enlightenment.

In distant times, legend has it that the great voyaging canoes from Tahiti and other islands would be guided to a safe landing on Hawaii's shores from the lamps and torches lit by the kukui. Candlenut oil is also used for preserving wood, tattooing, and painting. Polished kukui nuts strung into a lei are given as a special gift of love and *aloha*.

The ancient people of Hawaii were among the most resourceful of their time. They knew how to care for things that would, in time, care for them. Embedded within the aloha spirit is a wisdom way—"may we be guiding lights for one another."

At the age of four, my beloved daughter-in-law, Kalei, began learning the ancient Hawaiian custom of hula, which continued throughout her formative years. Her grandmother, Tutu Mary, was her teacher and guiding light in all her endeavors. When my grandson, Robert James, was born, I arrived to find Tutu Mary embracing him and softly singing his Hawaiian name: "Keaka Mai kalani…."

Tutu Mary translated our grandson's name for me. She smiled and said, "The light of the heavens, brightly shining with splendor as it rises in the morning light."

When that grandson was nearly age four, he called me early one morning. Surprised to hear his voice, I said, "Are you just waking up… isn't it still dark outside?" He emphatically replied, "No, Grandma Geri, the sun just hasn't come over the mountain yet!"

Synchronicities Abound

Hawaiian elders' wisdom teaches that synchronicities abound; premonitions and intuitive wisdom are a feature of daily life. In Hawaii's long tradition of oral poetry, there is always a story within the story. Elders teach with the murmur of the ocean in the background; "talking story" is a way of life.

Tutu is a respectful Hawaiian word for an elder, wise teacher, or grandparent. Sharing the hard-won wisdom of a lifetime is a task Tutu Mary takes seriously. When she shares stories of her ancestors, I am deeply honored. Singing in her melodious Hawaiian language while strumming a ukulele has been her customary way of greeting me when I arrive. She sings from the heart. Every breath and every word reveal her loving aloha spirit.

In traditional Hawaiian families, you meet, you eat, you tell stories, you listen. Above all, you listen. It is the Hawaiian way.

When my grandson was just a few months old, Tutu Mary began feeding him *poi* as she sang to him in the early morning. I learned that poi comes from taro—a bulbous, potato-like root that has been a dietary staple for centuries.

Taro is regarded as an ancestor. Its broad triangular leaves are lifted by a stem called the *Ha* which is also the Hawaiian word for breath—so that each stem is an umbilicus joining the plant world and the human world, a looping journey of open-ended searches and fortunate meetings.

Tutu in her native tongue—Hawaii's soft flowing language—nurtures and nourishes the grandchildren and great-grandchildren with the love and devotion of ancient ways. Tutu Mary lives her legacy—demonstrating generativity in action.

May we all be lights for one another!

"If a child is to keep alive
his inborn sense of wonder,
he needs the companionship
of at least one adult
who can share it,
rediscovering with him
the joy, excitement, and mystery
of the world we live in."

—RACHEL CARSON

"A hundred years from now
it will not matter
what my bank account was,
the sort of house I lived in,
or the kind of car I drove...
but the world may be different
because I was important
in the life of a child."

—FOREST E. WITCRAFT

Reflections:

Nine
Look Beyond Appearances

> "When living out from the center of Being,
> you are untouched and nothing acts upon you
> because you do not react
> to the world of appearances."

JOEL GOLDSMITH

Joel Goldsmith (1892-1964) is frequently referred to as a "mystical wayshower." Contemporary authors Eckhart Tolle and Wayne Dyer often cite Goldsmith's influence on their work.

Eckhart Tolle stated:

A new generation of mature seekers, receptive to spiritual truth, is now discovering Joel Goldsmith's teachings, which have lost none of their relevance and power. I foresee that those teachings will reach and impact more people in the twenty-first century than during his lifetime. Joel Goldsmith's profoundly inspiring books represent a vital contribution to the spiritual awakening of humanity.

Wayne Dyer tells audiences that for inspiration he keeps a photograph of Joel Goldsmith on his desk as he writes.

A Shift in Consciousness

I discovered a tremendous shift occurring in my own life on all levels—personal, professional, and spiritual—in the mid-1980s. When I came upon the written works of Joel Goldsmith, I was intrigued by his invitation to move into another level of conscious awareness—to see through the "appearances of this world." Soon thereafter, I discovered that Goldsmith audiotapes were played for a small group who met in silence every Thursday evening just a couple of miles from my home. When a neighbor mentioned the possibility of hearing such recordings, I was curious. By then, I had read many of Goldsmith's books but had never heard his voice. Eager to expand my awareness, I began to attend those weekly listening sessions. Each time I attended one of the gatherings, I sensed an atmosphere of calm that momentarily lifted me out of the chaos and challenges of everyday life. Like every other attendee, I entered in silence and left in silence. I discussed the experience with no one.

I began to feel a profound sense of peace. I certainly did not understand what was happening but I was eager to explore this new terrain.

A Contemplative Life

About that time, another teacher appeared in my life by coincidence. (I was beginning to see, however, that there are really no coincidences!) One evening, Bee Culver dropped by my home with a mutual friend for a cup of tea. Bee, a tall, gracious white-haired woman, sipped her chamomile tea and expressed interest in my work in gerontology. As she scanned my bookshelves, she noticed some of Joel Goldsmith's books tucked in among my collection of books on health and aging. Almost immediately, we were conversing with an openness of friends who had known each other forever.

Then my newfound friend shared an experience that caused me to gasp in astonishment. Over a decade earlier, Bee and her husband were rushing toward their car during a fierce rainstorm in Seattle when suddenly he reached down into a gutter and fished out a paperback book, shook it off, and handed it to her. She thought it rather strange but rather than protest, she accepted the soggy book and dropped it beneath her feet on the passenger side of the car. They drove home in silence, barely able to see the road through the pelting rain.

As they approached their modest dwelling in North Seattle, the storm's toll was everywhere. Branches from the majestic oak trees lay strewn across the lawn and streetlights were out. Wanting nothing more than to get inside and light the fireplace, Bee chose to appease her husband by carrying that squishy book inside. She tossed it under a heating vent thinking it would likely dry out or crumble. "In either case," she thought, "I will discard it later."

Little did Bee anticipate the impact of that rain-soaked book. "After about two days, I noticed the title, *The Contemplative Life* by Joel Goldsmith, and I began reading. Geri, I stayed up all night reading. Suddenly I felt a flash of light— yes, yes, this is what I have always known I was seeking. But no one had ever spoken to me about contemplation in this way." And, she softly added, "That was the beginning of a feeling of peace and serenity I never dreamed possible."

Bee truly radiated peace. We remained close friends until her passing at age 91. Over the years, I saw her weather circumstances that would have devastated most. The sudden death of her youngest son, Jack, was a painful blow. Jack was jogging to his son's soccer game when he fell from an overpass onto the highway below. He died just as Bee reached the hospital in Olympia, Washington to see what she described as "my youngest son's broken body." In the midst of her profound grief, Bee knew that Jack was more than his body.

Just a few months after Jack's death, I saw Bee consoling women whose children had died. Younger women seemed to gravitate toward her for counsel and guidance. Individuals she had never seen before approached her and poured out their hearts. She shone light that people of all ages seemed to recognize. Bee was a beholder of peace and serenity, but she rarely spoke of the Goldsmith works—sometimes called Infinite Way teachings—unless specifically asked.

Shortly before her passing, Bee told me that she wanted to give me her collection of Joel Goldsmith books. Now I have a treasure trove with her handwritten notes in nearly all of them. Bee was a wayshower; she taught others by her gentle demeanor and unconditional acceptance. I feel her presence each time I open one of those books.

Transcending Age through Contemplative Living

Virginia Stephenson, one of Joel Goldsmith's original students, is also my dear friend and teacher. Now in her mid-90s, Virginia resides in Hawaii, having traveled extensively to share the essence of Goldsmith's work for more than four decades.

Shortly before his death in 1964, Joel Goldsmith designated five teachers, all of whom had been his longtime students, to carry on his work. Virginia is one of those five. I invariably gain new insights through correspondence and conversations with her. Over the years, she has patiently answered even the most simplistic questions I have posed.

Through such illuminated wayshowers as Virginia and Bee, I have come to view growing older (in calendar years) as an opportunity to grow in spiritual meaningfulness. Virginia's ageless and gracious countenance is a vivid reminder that opportunities for growth never end. On a recent occasion I asked, "Virginia, could we talk about some of your ideas and some of the teachings that led you to such a joyful approach to aging?"

"Maturing—that is the word," Virginia responded. "The word *aging* never sounds right to me. The unfolding of consciousness is what takes place when we live fully. As youngsters, we explore the physical world and everything around us in the outer world. As time goes by, we become more interested in intellectual things. But there comes a time when we begin to inquire— is there not something more than just the physical and intellectual? Is there not something else? We feel that there must be another dimension. We can almost touch it, but we do not really know what it is."

I asked: "How can we access this other 'dimension' that you speak of?"

Virginia answered without hesitation: "We learn to meditate. We start to look within ourselves for the treasure we have, the treasure of inner peace. A quiet walk, an appreciation of nature, and a sense of gratitude for the good we have already received enables us to be receptive to this new dimension of unconditional Love." Then she added poetically, "We enter within to the silence of our own being—this *inner resort.*"

Virginia reminded me that when we find this "centering" place, we quite naturally become more tranquil. She said, "We have an inner resort that is the most refreshing, renewing, and restoring activity you can ever imagine. All the health spas, all the massages, all the long hours of sleep cannot renew you as much as 10 seconds of touching that inner resort of Love."

Accessing Your Inner Resort

When I asked Virginia to tell me more about accessing that inner resort, she said, "I think of a resort as a place where you rest your mind, where you stop taking thought about tomorrow or about yesterday, and you focus on the present moment. You rest from judging the appearance world." She added, "The inner resort is a place of peace and harmony."

Then Virginia briefly referred to the Eastern teachings: "The word *darshan* signifies inner peace. When you come into the presence of someone who is peaceful, you feel it."

I commented that I had often seen people drawn to my dear friend Bee, and that I felt she embodied darshan. "Oh, yes, Geri," Virginia said, "when you come into the presence of someone who does not judge you or criticize you but recognizes that you, too, have this inner resort, you are pulled into that quiet peaceful atmosphere. That is practicing the presence of Love."

Bee demonstrated kindness and peaceful qualities beyond measure; she introduced me to the essence of these words attributed to Lao Tzu:

Empty your mind of all thoughts.
Let your heart be at peace.
Watch the turmoil of beings,
But contemplate their return.

Each separate being in the universe
Returns to the common source.
Returning to the source is serenity.

If you don't realize the source,
You stumble in confusion and sorrow.
When you realize where you come from,
You naturally become tolerant,
Disinterested, amused,
Kindhearted as a grandmother,
Dignified as a king.
Immersed in the wonder of the Tao,
You can deal with whatever life brings you,
And when death comes you are ready.

"If the doors of perception
were cleansed,
everything would appear...
as it is,
infinite."

—WILLIAM BLAKE

"Stillness speaks. "

—ECKHART TOLLE

"Change the way
you look at things...
the things you look at
will change."

—WAYNE DYER

Reflections:

Ten
Cultivate Peace, Love, and Friendship

"Peace that passes understanding
can be reached only by compassion.
This is the ideal that must illumine,
from the very center,
all our efforts to bring a better life
to our world, within our own country,
and in the farthest reaches of the planet."

—R. SARGENT SHRIVER

"He changed my life," Bill Moyers emphatically stated at a reunion in Washington, D.C. honoring R. Sargent Shriver, founding director of the Peace Corps. Moyers, the broadcast journalist, is famous for his eloquent and incisive interviews on public television. He was also the deputy director of the Peace Corps at its inception.

In his tribute, Moyers reeled off movements that Shriver and his wife, Eunice Kennedy Shriver inspired: Peace Corps, Head Start, Vista, Job Corps, Community Action, Upward Bound, Foster Grandparents, Special Olympics. Moyers reminded us that Shriver lived his life with the certainty that it's what we do to serve, to help, and to care for our fellow human beings that counts in the long run.

I could also say that Shriver changed my life. My Peace Corps experience in Bolivia continues to impact my journey to this day. Now, more than 50 years later, I'm in regular contact by phone and email with my Bolivian friends and "family." I've returned to Sucre several times over the past decades as I've been invited to collaborate on international health consulting assignments in the region.

Among my extended family there are two precious young girls: One is named Pilar Geri; the other, Geri Estefania. My Bolivian friends have gifted and blessed me with their generous spirit in innumerable ways. Gratitude is forever embedded in my heart.

I regard the Peace Corps experience as a pivotal event in my life. Shriver reminded us as we departed for our countries of service that, in essence, all of us are members of the same great human endeavor and that our tents are merely pitched on different grounds. Shriver cautioned us to "go abroad, aware that the only change that really matters must come from within."

And he told us, "You need to realize the world is home to all." Furthermore, "You are to bring the world back home to share what you learned with our fellow citizens." Quite an assignment for a 22 year old!

Those early Peace Corps experiences continue to impact my beliefs and attitudes. I know they've been my springboard for exploring purposeful and meaningful aging!

We Give Thanks

As I sorted through stacks of paper after presenting a seminar for health care providers in Washington State, I came upon a handwritten note. To this day, I have no idea who left it, but the essence of a message embedded in that note is:

> We give thanks
> Thanks a million times over
> For those people, those rare,
> Precious, marvelous people
> Who have found a secret place
> And pitched their tents there.
> Those who dwell in attitudes
> Of hope and confidence,

Who reach across rather than down,
Those people whose presence
Always leaves us
Feeling better about ourselves.
We give thanks for these
Loving people,
Beacons for the unfoldment of Love.

I invite you to ponder on the significance of becoming a beacon in our world today. People everywhere are hungry for a message of hope, a message that allows us to embrace one another with understanding and acceptance instead of fear and mistrust. There is a great longing for the peace, the justice, and the dignity that are the birthright of all.

Since those formative years in Bolivia and Puerto Rico, I've had the opportunity to serve as an international health consultant in many parts of the world. Each assignment has brought lessons on its wing. I distinctly recall a stopover in Washington, D.C. as I was traveling to Kenya and Uganda, where I'd been invited to participate in global health work some years ago. Imagine my astonishment to find this message on my pillow at an inn—right in the heart of our nation's capital:

In ancient times, there was a prayer for
"The Stranger within Our Gate."
Because this hotel is a human institution
to serve people, and not solely a money-making

organization, we hope that you will be granted
peace and rest while you are under our roof.
May this room and hotel be your "second" home.
May those you love be near you in thoughts and dreams.

May the business that brought you our way prosper. May
every call you make and every message you receive add
to your joy. When you leave, may your journey be safe.

We are all travelers. From "birth 'til death" we travel
between eternities. May these days be pleasant for you,
profitable for society, helpful for those you meet, and a
joy to those who know and love you best.

I carry that poignant message wherever I go. Since that day my work has taken me to other countries in Africa as well as Central and South America, the Caribbean, Asia, Australia, and New Zealand.

Everywhere I travel, I see how our lives are interconnected. All of us have dreams and hopes and we seek meaning and purpose regardless of circumstances or age or geography.

Recently, I came upon my notes from a meeting with a group of healthcare providers in Mombasa, Kenya dated August 27, 1987. I wrote that the health division supervisors had completed a training needs assessment and were now preparing an in-service training plan for all health workers in the community health education program. My notes said "good needs assessment; organizing meeting for all directors next week to analyze results and develop an implementation strategy for training." All this was a standard part of my work assignment. I loved it.

Tucked into the back cover of my journal I noticed some notes I'd jotted to myself on that August day:

> Home is where your heart is…
> Be at home here… Now
> Move with assurance.
> Awaken with a song in your heart.
> Connect with Nature.
> Remember your Family extends to the World Community.
> Love dissolves all differences. May you always feel its warmth and protection directly from Source.

Turtles for Peace

I'm honored to be a lifetime member of the Viktor Frankl Institute of Logotherapy; I've presented my work at several of the biennial World Congresses. Upon completing an afternoon workshop on global aging at a World Congress that convened in Dallas, Texas, a silver-haired gentleman made his way slowly to the front of the room and offered me a gift—a tiny turtle carved from rose quartz that he carried in a tan leather bag. He said simply, "I cannot travel far these days so I give these turtles to people who will take them wherever they go in the world."

I marveled at the beauty of the rose quartz and thanked the gentleman, Mr. Bob Eckstrom, for the lovely gift.

He added "These turtles are making their way around the world slowly but in good time." Then he quietly stated, "I gave one to Archbishop Desmond Tutu. I call them Turtles for Peace."

That Turtle for Peace reminds me each day that all of us are called to break from our shells of fear and to birth a more soulful way of being. We are invited to create a more harmonious way to live and to open our hearts to unfold-ment. Precious gifts come to us in most unexpected ways, seen and unseen.

Turtles are found on every continent of the world. In South America, the Amazon people believe that the turtle is resourceful and knows how to emerge safely and victori-ously out of any challenging circumstances. That gentleman in Texas is gently reminding us through his Turtles for Peace that we are called to be part of a planetary shift, one that is calling each of us to a purposeful and significant life.

"To pray for the world
means to look out
as if seeing this globe
in front of you,
and feel your love
going out around it....
Hold that globe
in a whole armful of love,
understanding
and forgiveness....
Never think of victories,
think of Peace."

—JOEL GOLDSMITH

Reflections:

Acknowledgments

"The best and most beautiful things in the world cannot be seen or even touched... They must be felt with the heart."

—HELEN KELLER

Heartfelt thanks to all my teachers and to my "global family" who have awakened me to a path of purpose and meaning. Students, colleagues,friends, family, neighbors and scores of "persons in the street" have taught valuable lessons that I gratefully acknowledge. Each new day has held a lesson— though often recognized only in retrospect.

Drs. Robert and Dorothy Barnes and Dr. Ann Graber and the International Board of Directors of the Viktor Frankl Institute of Logotherapy have embraced my global work. I am indeed grateful for the honor of being a Lifetime Member of the Institute and also for the privilege of presenting my work at several biennial World Congresses of the Institute.

Special thanks to my editors, Charles McLafferty and Kate Robinson, whose genuine interest in my words has helped me beyond measure. Charles has studied the works of Viktor Frankl in depth and he shares my profound respect for Frankl's legacy and its relevance to today's world. Both Charles' and Kate's professional approach to editing makes writing a joyful experience.

Mil gracias to Roberto Burdman for his design of the book cover and for all the years of understanding my exploration of "pathways to meaningful aging" while motivating me on this journey.

Mahalo to Sam Horn, author and former Emcee of the Maui Writers Conference, for recognizing the value of my work and especially for encouraging me to "write on!" Sam's gifts of perceptive listening and crystallizing ideas are remembered often.

To my husband, Roberto, and to our sons, Robert Peter and Ethan David… thank you from the bottom of my heart… Grace and Gratitude…

Geri Marr Burdman
June, 2015

References and Related Readings

Allende, Isabel. *Paula*. New York: Harper Perennial, 2013

Angelou, Maya. *Even the Stars Look Lonesome*. New York: Random House, 1997

Atchley, Robert. *Spirituality and Aging*. Baltimore: Johns Hopkins University Press, 2009

Baldwin, Cristina. *Storycatcher*. Novato, CA: World Library, 2005

Barks, Coleman. *A Year with Rumi*. San Francisco: HarperCollins, 2006

Bateson, Mary Catherine. *Composing a Further Life: The Age of Active Wisdom*. New York: Knopf, 2010

Benson, Herbert. *Timeless Healing*. New York: Fireside, 1997

Bonanno, George A. *The Other Side of Sadness: What the New Science of Bereavement Tells Us about Life After Loss*. New York: Basic Books, 2009

Brokaw, Tom. *The Great Generation*. New York: Random House, 2004

Brokaw, Tom. *Boom! Voices of the Sixties*. New York: Random House, 2008

Brooks, David. *The Road to Character*. New York: Random House, 2015

Burdman, Geri Marr. *Healthful Aging*. Englewood Cliffs, NJ: Prentice-Hall, 1986

Burns, Ken. *The War: An Intimate Story, 1941-1945*. New York: Knopf, 2007

Butler, Robert. *Why Survive? Being Old in America*. Baltimore: The Johns Hopkins University Press, 2002

Butler, Robert. *The Longevity Revolution: The Benefits and Challenges of Living a Long Life*. New York: PublicAffairs, 2008

Byock, Ira. *The Best Care Possible*. New York: Penguin Group, 2012

Byock, Ira. *The Four Things that Matter Most* (10th ed.). New York: Atria, 2014

Campbell, Joseph. *Hero with a Thousand Faces*. Novato, CA: New World, 2008 (originally published 1949)

Carson, Rachel. *Silent Spring*. New York: Houghton Mifflin, 1962

Chittester, Joan. *The Gift of Years*. Katonah, NY: BlueBridge Publishing, 2010

Chopra, Deepak. *Peace is the Way*. New York: Random House, 2005

Dyer, Wayne. *Change Your Thoughts—Change Your life: Living the Wisdom of the Tao*. Carlsbad, CA: Hay House, 2007

Erikson, Erik and Joan. *The Life Cycle Completed*. New York: W. W. Norton, 1997

Frankl, Viktor. *The Doctor and the Soul*. New York: Second Vintage Books, 1986

Frankl, Viktor. *Man's Search for Ultimate Meaning*. New York: Basic Books, 2000

Frankl, Viktor. *Recollections. An Autobiography*. New York: Perseus, 2000

Frankl, Viktor. *The Unheard Cry for Meaning*. New York: Perseus, 2000

Frankl, Viktor. *Man's Search for Meaning*. Boston: Beacon Press, 2006

Gawande, Atul. *Being Mortal: Medicine and what Matters in the End*. New York: Henry Holt, 2014

Ghandi, Arun. *Legacy of Love: My Education in the Path of Nonviolence*. Wauconda, IL: Ghandi Worldwide Education Institute, 2009

Gilbert, Daniel. *Stumbling on Happiness*. New York: Random House, 2007

Goldsmith, Joel. *A Parenthesis in Eternity*. San Francisco: HarperOne, 1986

Goldsmith, Joel. *The Art of Meditation*. San Francisco: HarperOne, 1990

Goldsmith, Joel. *The Thunder of Silence*. New York: HarperCollins, 1993

Goldsmith, Joel. *The Contemplative Life*. New York: Carol Publishing Group, 1994

Goldsmith Joel. *The Heart of Mysticism*. Camarillo, CA: Devross, 2007

Graber, Ann. *Viktor Frankl's Logotherapy: Method of Choice in Ecumenical Pastoral Psychology*. Lima, OH: Wyndham Hall Press, 2004

Graber, Ann. *The Journey Home: Preparing for Life's Ultimate Adventure*. Birmingham, AL: Purpose Research, 2009

Horn, Sam. *Got Your Attention?* San Francisco, CA: Berrett Koehler, 2015

Isay, David, (Ed). *Listening is an Act of Love: A Celebration of American Lives from the Story Corps Project*. New York: Penguin Press, 2007

Jampolsky, Jerry. *Love is Letting Go of Fear*. Millbrae, CA: Celestial Arts, 1979

Kabat-Zinn, Jon. *Arriving at Your Own Door: 108 Lessons in Mindfulness*. New York: Hyperion, 2007

Kimble, Melvin. *Aging, Spirituality, and Religion*. Minneapolis: Fortress Press, 2002

Klingberg, Haddon, Jr. *When Life Calls Out to Us: The Love and Lifework of Viktor and Elly Frankl*. New York: Doubleday, 2001

Kornfield, Jack. *The Wise Heart*. New York: Bantam Dell, 2008

Kristoff, Nicholas and Sheryl WuDunn. *A Path Appears*. New York: Knopf, 2014

Kübler-Ross, Elisabeth. *Death, the Final Stage of Growth*. Englewood Cliffs, NJ: Prentice-Hall, 1975

Langer, Ellen. *Counterclockwise: Mindful Health and the Power of Possibility*. New York: Ballantine Books, 2009

Lear, Linda. *Rachel Carson: Witness for Nature*. New York: Houghton-Mifflin Harcourt, 1997

Leider, Richard. *The Power of Purpose: Find Meaning, Live Longer, Better* (2nd ed.). San Francisco: Berrett-Koehler, 2008

Lesser, Elizabeth. *Broken Open: How Difficult Times Can Help Us Grow*. New York: Villard Books, 2005

Luskin, Fredrick. *Forgive for Good*. New York: HarperCollins, 2004

Moody, Harry and David Carroll. *The Five Stages of Soul*. New York: Doubleday, 1999

Moyers, Bill. *Fooling with Words: A Celebration of Poets and their Craft*. New York: Perennial, 2001

Nugent, Joy. *As Good as Good-Byes Get: A Window into Death and Dying*. Pittsburg: Dorrance Publishing, 2015

Pattakos, Alex. *Prisoners of our Thoughts: Viktor Frankl's Principles for Discovering Meaning in Life and Work*. San Francisco: Berrett-Koehler, 2004

Pevny, Ron. *Conscious Living, Conscious Aging*. New York: Atria, 2014

Pizer, Marjorie. *Selected Poems*. Sydney: Pinchgut Press, 1984

Sarton, May. *Coming into Eighty: Poems*. New York: W. W. Norton, 1994

Schacter-Shalomi, Zalman and Ronald Miller. *From Age-ing to Sage-ing: A Profound New Vision of Growing Older*. New York: Warner Books, 1997

Schiltz, Marilyn. *Living Deeply*. Oakland: New Harbinger, 2008

Shriver, Maria. *Just Who Will You Be?* New York: Hyperion, 2008

Shriver, Mark. *A Good Man: Rediscovering my Father, Sargent Shriver*. New York: Henry Holt, 2012

Shriver, Sargent. *Point of the Lance*. New York: Harper and Row, 1964

Sorenson, Ted. *Counselor: A Life at the Edge of History*. New York: HarperCollins, 2008

Southwick, Steven and Dennis Charney. *Resilience*. New York: Cambridge University Press, 2012

Stephenson, John. *The Fullness of Joy: A Spiritual Guide to the Paradise Within*. Camarillo, CA: DeVorss & Company, 2012

Stephenson, Virginia. *Genesis. Awakening from the Dream.* Atlanta: Acropolis Books, 1997

Thomas, William. *What are Old People For? How Elders Will Save the World*. Acton, MA: Vanderwyk & Burnham, 2007

Tolle, Eckhart. *Stillness Speaks*. Novato, CA: New World Library, 2003

Toms, Justine. *Simple Pleasures: Finding Grace in a Chaotic World*. Charlottesville, VA: Hampton Roads Publishing, 2008

Tutu, Desmond. *No Future without Forgiveness*. New York: Doubleday, 2000

Tutu, Desmond and Mpho Tutu. *The Book of Forgiving: The Four-fold Path for Healing Ourselves and Our World*. New York: HarperCollins, 2015.

Williams, Margery. *The Velveteen Rabbit*. Available at the URL: www.gutenberg.org/ebooks/11757. Originally published 1922

Williamson, Marianne. *The Age of Miracles*. Carlsbad: CA: Hay House, 2008

Zukov, Gary. *Soul to Soul: Communications from the Heart*. New York: Free Press, 2007

About the Author

Geri Marr Burdman is a health promotion and gerontology specialist who offers a unique interdisciplinary and transcultural perspective on the integration of mind-body-spirit.

After earning her Ph.D. from the University of Oregon, Geri Marr Burdman has served on the faculties of Case Western Reserve University, the University of Oregon, and the University of Washington. Her books and educational seminars focus on promoting quality and dignity throughout the lifespan. She has presented her work in many parts of the world including Africa, Asia, Australia, New Zealand, Europe, the Caribbean, Central and South America as well as Canada and the USA. Geri was among the first Peace Corps Volunteers to serve in Bolivia.

Geri Marr Burdman met Dr. Viktor Frankl, founder of Logotherapy and author of *Man's Search for Meaning* in Puerto Rico in the late 1960s. Profoundly impacted by Frankl's unwavering conviction that the motivating force behind all human behavior is a pursuit of meaning, Geri actively promotes the principles of Logotherapy in her work. She is a Lifetime Member of the Viktor Frankl Institute of Logotherapy.

Geri is the founder of GeroWise® International (www.gero-wise.com). Currently she divides her time between Washington State and Arizona.

Dear Reader,

Thank you for your interest in our work. We welcome your comments and feedback.

For information and to order books, please contact:

GeroWise® Books

Division of GeroWise® International
308 East Goodwin Street
Prescott, AZ 86303 USA

gerimar@mindspring.com
www.gerowise.com

CPSIA information can be obtained
at www.ICGtesting.com
Printed in the USA
FSOW03n1002110815
9584FS